# GOOD TIME YOGA
## for the
# NOT-SO-YOUNG

Marianna Halasz

T0149349

**BALBOA.**
PRESS
A DIVISION OF HAY HOUSE

Balboa Press books may be ordered through booksellers or by contacting:

Balboa Press
A Division of Hay House
1663 Liberty Drive
Bloomington, IN 47403
www.balboapress.com.au
1 (877) 407-4847

Print information available on the last page.

ISBN: 978-1-5043-1853-2 (sc)
ISBN: 978-1-5043-1854-9 (e)

Balboa Press rev. date: 07/09/2019

# RECOMMENDATION

At the end of a busy day consulting in my GP practice, it is good to have something to look forward to and a deadline, so I finish on time and get to the weekly yoga class.

Marianna Halasz began yoga classes in Gundagai in 2003 and I was one of the first to attend. Her passion for yoga and her expertise were on display in every class.

One mantra she would say to us most weeks, is that the exercises and poses may seem easy but if you think about what you are doing and don't let your mind wander it will be twice as beneficial. In other words, leave the problems of the day and the world outside the yoga room.

This took me sometime to achieve but I eventually managed this most of the time. Marianna was an early advocate of Mindfulness.

Another mantra she often made in her very Hungarian accent was "just do what you can do, but do it correctly". This was so each person could gain maximum personal benefit without causing themselves any injury. "Next week you will be able to do a bit more."

A good night's sleep always followed Marianna's yoga classes as the body had been put through many restorative moves and the mind had achieved a degree of relaxation. Both are good reasons that I continue to go to yoga classes each week and find some time each day for a little yoga.

Over the years I have recommended yoga to many of my patients and many of them still attend the classes regularly and quite a few have thanked me for the advice.

Congratulations Marianna on your book and thank you for sharing your expertise with me and the people of Gundagai.

Virginia Wrice MBBS (Hons) FACRRM FRACGP

# ACKNOWLEDGEMENTS

I would like to express my greatest gratitude and love to the following people.

I appreciate the encouragement provided by *Peggy Elliott*, the Manageress of Gundagai Neighbourhood Centre for allowing me to start a class of "Good time Yoga". The class for the students was made a little easier by sitting and standing. Since this Yoga was considered as helpful and beneficial for the "not so young" generation, the participants were only charged a few dollars per lesson. It became more and more popular as the years followed.

My friend *Gina Keogh* helped in many ways with the editing and proof reading. She donated selflessly her time and experience for the fulfilment of this presentation.

Many thanks to *Lena Elphick* for editing, taking the photographs and arranging them in the book. She also designed the front cover and generously donated her expertise and technical knowledge.

*Robyn Hockey* deserves my full admiration for modelling and putting up with the inconvenience of posing for many hours in order for the photographs to be correct.

I would also like to thank *Dr Virginia Wrice* who practices yoga herself. She has recommended many of her *not so young patients* to join the "Good time Yoga" classes.

Finally, thanks to *Balboa Publisher* for the polite and professional help by its employees to produce the final product.

I would like to extend my heartfelt gratitude to all my students who allowed me to share my experience as a Yoga instructor in the past 25 years.

I hope that the people who practice the Yoga recommended in my book, will make themselves and the world a little better than it was before.

# CONTENTS

# (HAPTER 1

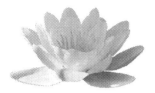

## Introduction

Whatever age you are, it is never too late to learn new things.

We only have one body in this lifetime. In order to make our body serve us better, we should look after it the best we can. Whilst growing up, we are first influenced by our parents, and then we receive an education in school. We are taught how important it is to have a profession in order to gain employment. We all want a family and work to acquire all the possessions and gadgets that make our lives more comfortable. We look after all of our things and also want to have better lives and strive to serve society.

There are no coincidences in life. There is a reason why you found this book, or rather why this book found you. There are no causes without effect. This book is the result, the effect caused by your own actions in your life. There's a reason you are reading this text; this book was written for you, with you in mind.

There may be something you are meant to learn from this book, or perhaps you have chosen to buy it for someone who could benefit from the exercises. You are never too old to rearrange the knowledge you have gained through exercise and changing your lifestyle. The improvements to your body and mind can be achieved by using simple tools.

People have busy lives and often forget how to look after themselves. In their younger days, some may have taken part in physical activity: sports, athletics, perhaps ballet or gymnastics. Due to different circumstances or injuries, they stopped doing their exercise. Others succumbed to boredom or quit simply because they're no longer young.

One of the most important requirements for everyone is the ability to change. Change is the only thing that is permanent in our lives.

To remain young, not only bodily but mentally and, dare I say, spiritually, we have to keep our bodies and minds supple, flexible, and healthy. The most important question concerns our ability to retain (or regain) our health. How can we achieve this easily, and how can we adjust our lifestyles to make these changes?

The answer is simple: You become young in mind and spirit if you practise yoga.

More than five hundred years before the birth of Christ, the Greek philosopher Heraclitus said, "You cannot step into the same river twice, because the water runs and changes and nothing stands still."

This statement is true even today. We have to adapt ourselves to change. Taking advantage of the development of all the technical and scientific discoveries, we must adopt a new way of thinking and living.

We can achieve health using a simple tool. Practising yoga can be done at any time in our life, whether we are young or not so young any more. It keeps us healthier and younger.

Yoga is the union between the positive and negative energies in our body and mind. Unlike thirty or forty years ago, it is now accepted almost everywhere in the world.

*Marianna Halasz*

Due to growing interest, health organisations started to research yoga. Initially, these organisations tried to prove that yoga was not able to achieve what it professed. Yoga experts claimed that it was a healthy method to improve one's life.

Researchers studying the physical exercises of hatha yoga found some revealing evidence while experimenting with meditators. The practitioners suffered fewer sicknesses and were healthier and more peaceful than the average person, who ignored or even ridiculed these practises. Silence followed the evidence for many years, until it was impossible to dispute the benefits of yoga.

The German philosopher Arthur Schopenhauer expressed his views like this: "Every great idea goes through three phases before it is accepted. In the first it is rejected, in the second it is ridiculed, and in the third it is held to be self-evident."

One of the most difficult things, as we are aging, is to change our mind and our point of view. For some reason, women all over the world are more receptive and more prepared to adapt to changes. The round Chinese symbol of energy symbolises the male Yang and the female Yin. The union represents opposites, such as day and night.

For many reasons, more women practise tai chi and yoga than men. Both practises are slow and done meditatively. Gentle exercises tend to resonate with women's feminine side.

Ultimately, we are conditioned by our Westernised upbringing. It takes perseverance, energy, and money for our parents to educate us. Most of the education is correct. We all need guidance on how to live our life morally and physically. However, Western education also causes us to become stuck in our traditional views, as to what is right and what is wrong.

We mustn't forget that education does not end with our schooling. Learning is an ongoing process that lasts for as long as we live. Changing our minds about what we have learned in the past does not mean that we were taught incorrectly.

Changing our viewpoint simply means that we have taken our understanding to a different level. Nowadays, articles about yoga are common in newspapers, scientific journals, and women's magazines. The articles advise readers to practise yoga in order to improve their lives.

# CHAPTER 2

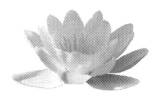

To exist in this world, we must follow four basic rules:

- breathe properly (more to follow)
- drink plenty of fresh water
- eat the right food
- move your body

The human body is designed and created for movement. Without any of the above-mentioned essentials, we cannot have a balanced healthy life.

Human beings have three ages:

1. Chronological age. This is based on the year, month, and day of birth. This cannot be changed.
2. Biological age. Flexibility and health changes from person to person. The health of two people of the same age, let's say fifty, can be different. One can be healthy, energetic, and contented, while the other is full of ailments, constantly complaining, bitter, and unhappy.
3. Psychological age. This reflects how well you feel and how old you feel.

Forty or even fifty years ago, many people viewed yoga as superstitious nonsense. As mentioned earlier, several years of experimenting has proven the benefits of yoga. Everyone can be changed dramatically through yoga exercises. It is not possible to change your chronological age; however, there are ways around it.

## We Can Change Our Biological Age

People are less flexible after forty years of age. There is no point in being upset or disappointed that you cannot do the things you did when you were younger. You should be happy that you gained plenty of experience in sport: running, dancing, doing gymnastics, or playing tennis or squash.

People who practise yoga exercises for a while recognise the benefits that yoga offers. You may even notice an improvement to your self-esteem.

If you practise yoga, you should give yourself the appreciation that you rightly deserve. If you do not appreciate yourself, no one else will. Also, it's never too late to change your way of thinking. It is healthy to open your mind when trying out something new and unusual.

Yoga will replace the need for energy that was required by the physical activities in your youth. If you do the yoga exercises recommended in this book, you may regain a healthy, balanced body, and you may also find contentment in your life.

It is important for you to feel good and psychologically young. Yoga practitioners learn how to make the necessary movements; they also learn how to breathe correctly. Breathing properly will change your whole personality. You will become more efficient and effective in your actions, and the positive influence will spread into your whole life.

## Being Young and Beautiful Is Not the Only Way to Be Happy

Happiness does not last for long. It can be measured in minutes and hours. Contentment is far more important; it can last a lifetime. To achieve contentment, you have to be grateful for what you have. If you are religious and want to develop spiritually, you should thank the universe for what you have. Gratitude will create contentment.

Earlier experiments into the process of aging were conducted on volunteer university students. The volunteers had to lie in a bed, and to prevent movement, their arms and legs were placed in tubes. In a couple of weeks their biological age was a lot older than their chronological age. When they returned to their normal lifestyles, the volunteers regained their actual age. The experiment proved how important it is to move our bodies.

Sooner or later, physically active people have to slow down. Age determines the body's capability. Yoga differs from physical exercise. It can be done by children, adults, those in middle age, and even people who are not so young.

Yoga can be practised by men and women in their eighties and even nineties. You have a much better chance of achieving that age if you have a healthy and a balanced body.

This book describes simple yoga exercises you can do in a group or on your own. The book is easy to take on your travels if you are staying in a hotel or motel. All you need is an armless chair and a space where you can stand and stretch your body. Loose and comfortable clothing is preferable.

**Important.** Ensure that the chair you use is not able to slip, as the movements may cause the chair to become unbalanced.

The exercises must not be hurried. You have to train yourself to do yoga slowly and consciously. You must keep your mind on each movement you make; breathing correctly is most important.

Yoga is designed to move your joints; consequently, ligaments, tendons, and muscles are exercised. Good health and flexibility will eventually affect your everyday actions. With a positive outlook and persistence, you will achieve some of your aims, whatever they may be, with better results.

Whether you are young or not-so-young, these slow and gentle movements can be practised safely by everyone. They will make your bones and muscles stronger and healthier; your whole body will feel better. The exercises can also prevent you from losing your balance and falling. They can protect you from future injures.

It is most important that you read all the information contained in this book. The yoga theory and physical descriptions will guide you along the way. Before beginning to practise yoga, you may want to discuss your intention with your doctor or physician. Your doctor should know what condition you are in and whether you are ready and able to do these exercises.

Most people are comfortable in choosing a traditional lifestyle. As creatures of habit, we become convinced that we are doing the right thing for ourselves, our families, and our society.

Deep within ourselves, perhaps without realising, we are afraid of changing. We tend to avoid the thought of learning and doing anything new. Yet we become tired and overworked or develop sicknesses simply because in our busy lifestyles, we forget to look after our own interests.

Women, in particular, are raised to think about others first. They tend to consider the problems of their children, husbands, relations, and friends before they take care of themselves.

*Marianna Halasz*

Historically, women have been oppressed, and society has controlled their decision making. In recent times, more women have been able to decide what they want to do with their own lives.

We cannot avoid aging. However, we can change our attitude towards aging. With yoga for the not-so-young, we can achieve a better outcome.

We exist only during this second. Every second on earth gives us the chance to change the way we think and act. We are all able to consider the possibilities of changing our attitudes and belief systems, if we want to achieve different outcomes in our lives.

# CHAPTER 3

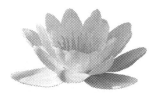

## Stress

Stress causes us to age more rapidly. We cannot avoid it in our lives. From the moment we are born, we are faced with struggle. Stress is caused by dwelling on our past misfortunes and anticipating future events that may go wrong.

It has been scientifically proven that by recalling past misfortunes or bad memories, our brains create harmful toxins. Even though we are aware of the fact that these things are not actually happening right now, our brain is unable to make this distinction.

We can learn from this scientific evidence by making an effort to live in the present. As observers looking at ourselves, we have the power to control our thoughts and actions.

Eckhart Tolle explained the ability to control and modify our lives in his book *The Power of Now.*

We live every moment of our life in the present. Every second, every minute, and every hour is a new beginning. We are constantly given the opportunity to change, to learn, and to grow, mentally and spiritually.

It does not matter how old you are. You will be able to do at least some of the yoga described in this book, and consequently, your health should improve along the way.

The most important thing to consider is, never underestimate the effectiveness of Good Time Yoga due to the apparent simplicity of the exercises. They are just as valid, important, and effective as the most complicated advanced hatha yoga postures. Yoga will make you feel years younger. You will be able to enjoy your life once more. You will be able do what you want, better and easier.

What's more, because you learn to balance your body with your mind and lifestyle, your way of thinking changes. You will also make better decisions for yourself in almost every situation.

Yoga will give you freedom, harmony, and suppleness of both your body and mind. These changes will happen gradually and slowly. The subtle development cannot be achieved in a week, but the changes in your body and mind are inevitable.

Yoga does not claim to act like an aspirin or a painkiller when you have a headache (however, some neck exercises can relieve tension headaches).

People who have meditated and practised yoga for a period of time feel up to twelve years younger biologically.

This claim has been proven by medical experiments. Practitioners of yoga are healthier and lead a more contented lifestyle; last but not least, their sex life is improved.

You might be sceptical after reading all these wonderful promises offered by yoga. The proof of the pudding is in the tasting, as the saying goes. Try it for a short time; a month is a good trial period for you to enjoy all the benefits of this method.

You might ask, like so many people before you, why anyone in the Western world would try an exercise method that was developed in India over five thousand years ego. Surely, with all the technical and scientific development in Western civilisation, we should know better.

The answer to this is simple. Technical progress and inventions have also created countless illnesses through pollution and stress. Westerners suffer from their harried, stressful lifestyles.

Even though yoga began in India, it can be useful for everyone. The whole world has enjoyed the benefits of penicillin, discovered by the Australian Nobel laureate Howard Florey. Another Nobel laureate, Hungarian physiologist Albert Szentgyörgyi, introduced the therapeutic effects of vitamin C to the world. We should be grateful for the hundreds of therapeutic scientific discoveries that are used by the whole world. The science of yoga is among these beneficial practises.

This relaxed, peaceful method will provide you what it promises. It will bring peace, good health, and a longer, more enjoyable life.

While this sounds too simple to be effective, I can assure you that its simplicity will help you to become more flexible.

Additionally, your internal organs are stimulated by conscious breathing. This massage isn't possible through your everyday activity. Through the consciously activated motions, you are also rewiring your brain. The stimulation will serve your body and your mind.

# CHAPTER 4

Welcome to the most beneficial and exciting experience of your life.

Never compare yourself to anyone. Everyone is built differently. If you have attended yoga classes in the past, you may have noted that some people are more flexible than you. During Good Time Yoga, you should not take any notice of this. Alternately, you should not be proud of yourself if you are more flexible than others.

Yoga is not a competition.

You are doing yoga for yourself and nobody else.

You are the one who mainly benefits from the improvements.

This book was written for those who are ready to change, knowing that change is the only permanent thing in life. This book gives you an opportunity to change, learn, and improve your body to become healthier and more contented.

Yoga simply means union of body and mind. Some people think yoga is a complicated combination of exercises, that you have to make a pretzel out of yourself to gain a beautiful body in order to impress people around you; the time has come for them to change their way of thinking.

With the slow and simplified method described in this book, you can achieve a healthy body and inner beauty that will make you feel relaxed and peaceful. You do not need to master all the advanced moves meant for those who have practised yoga from a young age.

The simple form of yoga I advocate is as beneficial as hatha yoga, and it may be even better for some of you. Later on, I will explain why it is effective.

The effects achieved will produce results that will surprise you and anyone who comes into contact with you. Good Time Yoga can also help those who are already familiar with other types of yoga. It might lead them back to the more advanced types.

Gentle yoga is recommended for people suffering from sport injuries or recovering from some type of illness or an operation. It will help regain the flexibility of both the body and mind. Most importantly, this is a modified form of yoga designed for the not-so-young.

Yoga targets your body and mind, and it is balanced with correct breathing. It will make your body movements lighter and easier.

To experience the full-term benefits, the participants should give themselves some time and be patient when waiting to see the effectiveness of this method. Yoga is a slow worker. The subtle changes to the body and mind take time to be apparent.

It takes time before the practitioners feel the benefits of yoga. Friends or relatives may notice the improvements first and comment on the changes of behaviour or their well-being.

All these claims may sound too improbable for some readers, especially those who are unfamiliar with yoga, but the simple exercises that are described in this book can do all that it promises.

*Marianna Halasz*

Everyone should enjoy the benefits of yoga, by doing what they can do without the pressure of impressing others.

When joining a yoga class, listen carefully to the instructor and observe whether she or he is sympathetic. A good teacher should have rapport and empathy with all of the students.

The prescribed exercises should be done preferably under the guidance of a well-trained yoga teacher. Participants tend to influence each other subconsciously, without realising this is happening. Gentle correction is always more effective than harsh criticism.

After a while, practitioners can do these routines in the privacy of their home. It is recommended that the exercises should be done regularly and preferably every day for at least twenty minutes. If it this is not possible, for whatever reason, the routine should be performed at least three or four times a week in the prescribed manner.

Yoga for the Not-So-Young participants learn how to

- breathe properly,
- do the different movements, and
- keep their mind on the exercise.

Breathing haphazardly during any exercise should be avoided. Busy people tend to have confusing thoughts involving their social lives, work, shopping, and other distractions.

The exercises are more effective and beneficial if you keep your mind on what you are doing whilst breathing properly. That is what makes a simple or complicated movement in your life yoga. This is the most important rule in order to achieve the best results.

Again, it should be emphasised that this method offers the best way to improve your general health and well-being. Your age and level of fitness do not matter. This gentle method helps you recover from injury or illness, and even people who are not so young will become more flexible.

It is important to look after your body's muscles and bones by making them stronger. Enhancing your balance can help you avoid bone-breaking falls.

Do your yoga exercises in order to enjoy them. You must have heard the phrase "No pain no gain." However, this point of view can work against you. Pain is a warning system designed to protect your body from further injury. Pain causes stress which consequently can lead to ill health.

I tell my students repeatedly, "Just do as much as you can. Never force your body." The moment you feel any discomfort or pain, it is a sign that you are doing something wrong.

The pain or discomfort in your body is actually telling you, "This is too much for me." Do whatever you can do with ease, and it will give you more satisfaction and better results. What you cannot do for the time being, you will achieve later, if you are persistent and follow the right instructions.

In the future, your body may surprise you. You can become more flexible, and these exercises will become easier as you progress. If you are stiff and suffer some soreness and discomfort after your first sessions, take heart in the fact that your body is responding to a new set of rules. Your body is simply trying to tell you, "This is completely unusual for me, and I don't like it. I don't like to move in this unfamiliar way."

Even people who exercise regularly notice that if they miss some lessons for a period of time, certain parts of their body will become stiff.

This stiffness and discomfort will disappear once yoga movements and stretches resume.

Be gently persistent until you get used to these new movements.

If you keep up the exercises, there will come a time when you will get used to doing yoga, and your body will miss the movements. Also, if initial discomfort dictates the terms, you have to decide who the boss is. Your body may not want to do new things, but you know that the yoga will be beneficial to you.

Most importantly, you must keep your mind on the exercise and breathe properly in order to make it yoga.

# CHAPTER 5

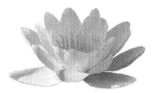

**Losing Weight**

Unlike strenuous exercise, yoga does not burn a lot of calories. Most people won't lose weight by doing yoga. Sometimes, fasting can work in weight loss. However, you should always discuss weight loss with your doctor first. Diets should be healthy and balanced in order to be beneficial.

I was most surprised when I first read about the importance of yoga when fasting.

My first reaction was, the body has to deal with the fact that the person is fasting, so why give it more problems?

When I looked into this question further, I learned that if we don't do any exercise or yoga while fasting, we will lose weight from body mass and bone density.

After most people practise yoga for a while, they appear to lose weight. However, if they stand on the scales, they will find that they haven't. This is because with the yoga practise, they have squeezed the fat out of the muscles. The muscles become longer stronger and slimmer. Muscle weighs almost the same as fat.

*Marianna Halasz*

# CHAPTER 6

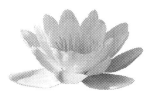

## Preparation

Do these warm-up exercises to start every session:

First and most importantly, you must ask your doctor if you are on certain medication that may clash with yoga. Blood pressure medications, for instance, can cause dizziness. Explain to your doctor that you want to try a simplified version of yoga.

Some doctors are not familiar with yoga. If your doctor agrees with your exercise plan, you must find the appropriate yoga teacher. As advised, do your lessons regularly. If you are familiar and have experienced yoga, do the exercises slowly by yourself.

Warming up exercises are most important. Let your body know you are ready to do yoga. Warming up is a wake-up call for your brain to be mindful. This usually happens without thinking about it. Keep your mind on whatever you are about to do. Your mind and brain will automatically send the necessary energy to your body in order to do the required exercise.

At the same time, listen to your body. The slightest discomfort or pain is a sign for you to stop and check the situation. Maybe you are making a wrong movement. It needs to be corrected by you or your yoga instructor. Or perhaps the pain is a warning that you have an injured body part that needs special attention. You may need some time to recover. If the pain persists, a visit to the doctor is essential.

## Basic Sitting Position for Good Time Yoga

Sit on an armless chair, with your back straight; do not lean on the back of the chair. Your head is an extension of your spine. Keep it in the normal position (the average human head weighs about one and a half a kilograms).

Your spine is designed to hold your head well balanced so that you don't feel its weight. At first, when people start doing yoga, they are tempted to move the head in different directions to the body.

This tends to happen especially during meditation or visualisation. There is a strong urge to bend the head forward and close the eyes. This may come from the act of being humble in church while listening and praying.

During yoga, your eyes should be open. Your eyes will determine if you are poised in a balanced position. Tilting the head, by bending it forward or backward, will damage the vertebrae in your neck. Over long periods, this could cause significant pain and damage. Therefore, it is very important to keep your head in the position that is required by the specific exercises you are about to do.

Please note: Ensure that the chair you use is not able to slip, as the movements may cause the chair to become unbalanced.

Maintaining balance is very important. The chair should be placed on a level surface. Wall-to-wall carpet is preferable to loose mats. If you have tiled or linoleum floors, ensure that the chair legs have a rubberised base that grips the floor's surface. Do not proceed with the exercises if the chair is liable to slip and slide.

Before starting the exercise, please remove your shoes. It would be better if you are barefooted, but you can wear non-slip socks.

## Preparing for the Exercises

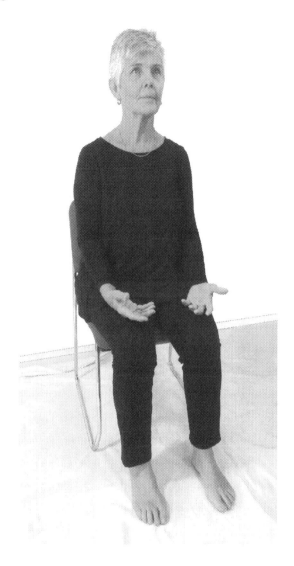

When sitting, hold your shoulders back as you push your chest forward. Your hands should be relaxing on your knees. Your palms can face down or both can be turned upward collecting prana (the Sanskrit word for universal energy). Look at a point in the opposite direction or lower your gaze looking at a point without focusing.

## Beginning Yoga

A yoga teacher begins a relaxation session by saying, "Take a few deep breaths, then relax your feet … your ankles … your calf muscles … your knees … your thighs … your hip joints. Make sure your back is straight and you breathe easily. Now relax your hands … your wrists … your fingers … your lower arms … your elbows … your upper arms. Relax all your neck muscles … all of your facial muscles … your jaw … your lips … your eyes … your forehead … your scalp. Feel your whole body relaxed, peaceful, and healthy."

The words should be repeated slowly. If you are alone, you should slowly start repeating the words in order to consciously slow down the whole body. Relax as much as possible, and think of the body part that is mentioned for relaxation.

*Marianna Halasz*

# CHAPTER 7

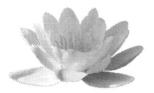

## Simple Meditation

To allow yourself to reach a relaxed state, your yoga teacher may read a short meditation text that will help you to further relax. If you are alone, you may prefer to sit quietly for a minute or so. It would be better if you do not close your eyes during this time.

Your brain may think that you want to go to sleep. That is not your aim at this point. Keep your eyes open, looking at a point but do not focus on it. Stay this way for a minute or as long as it feels comfortable for you. In this manner, you can meditate or make yourself relaxed anywhere you are. You may be sitting in the doctor's waiting room or a railway station, and nobody will know that you are meditating.

The best and easiest way to meditate is by watching your breath. This is a very simple and effective way to meditate. Basically, you centre your mind and body by paying attention to your breathing.

Remember that even whilst doing the simplest form of exercise, your whole body participates. When you are moving one part of your body, your leg, for example, you have to know how to hold your head and other parts of your body for the sake of balance.

When you have reached a calm state of relaxation, you are ready to learn the most important health promoting exercise, which is breathing properly.

This might sound strange, and some of you may think, *I have been breathing all my life since birth. What more can I learn from this?*

Now you should consider: Most of the time, we breathe haphazardly, without using the full capacity of our lungs. When working, doing house chores, or exercising, our attention is on the next thing we are supposed to do.

While participating in sports, we concentrate on watching the ball, anticipating when to kick it, hit it, or catch it. In our busyness, our breathing becomes haphazard and shallow.

Consequently, we use up the oxygen in our lungs and start gasping for air. Breathing the yoga way is healthier, and most importantly, we will be able to store up extra energy for future use. We have to keep mindful and pay full attention to the breathing exercises. After a while, healthy breathing becomes a normal habit, and you don't have to think about it.

# (HAPTER 8

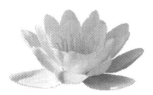

## Three Steps: Breathing the Yoga Way

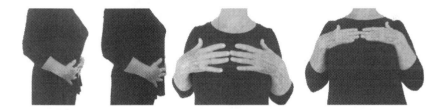

All conscious "breathing in" should happen through the nose. The nose is a very important organ. Its role is to filter the incoming air and warm the oxygen before it reaches the throat and lungs.

Sit, hold your upper body straight, and do not lean back on the chair. Your feet should be resting on the floor. Your head should be in the normal position and not bent in any direction. Keep your eyes open and look ahead at eye level or lower your gaze in a relaxed manner without focusing. Breathe easily.

Place both hands on your stomach, with the middle fingers gently touching. First, push your stomach muscles forward. When your stomach muscles are pushed forward, your lungs fill up with fresh air.

Think now of the middle part, your rib cage, as you breathe through your nose and feel your chest expanding and your fingertips move apart.

Next, fill up the top part of your lungs. When your lungs are full, and you feel you cannot fill them any further, hold your breath for three to five seconds.

Breathe out, pulling your stomach muscles in, and start emptying the middle part and the lower part by blowing out the air from your lungs through your slightly open mouth. Breathe out as much air as you can.

Holding the breath will fill up your lungs with oxygen and clear all those little crevices in the linings of your lungs. The oxygen gets rid of the accumulated unwanted residue from your lungs.

This may sound complicated, so here is the simplified version:

- To breathe in, push the stomach muscles forward.
- Fill up the lungs through the nostrils, and keep your lips closed.
- Breathe out through a slightly open mouth, and pull the stomach muscles in at the same time.

*Marianna Halasz*

## Breathing in and out of One Nostril at a Time

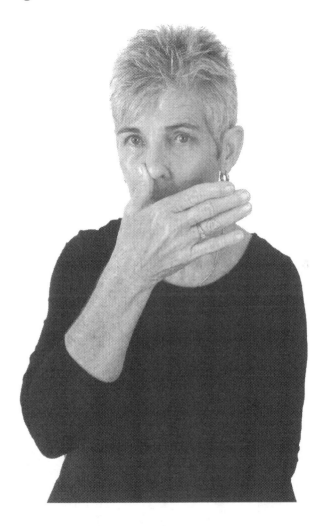

Sit in the basic yoga posture with the thumb of your right hand pushing in your right nostril. Inhale slowly on the left side (stomach, rib cage, top of your lungs), and hold your breath for a while before exhaling slowly on the same side. Change fingers of the right hand by placing your middle finger on your left nostril. Take a long breath in and hold it for a while before breathing out from the left side. Repeat this procedure four or five times.

# CHAPTER 9

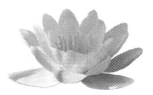

**Feet and Hand Warming Exercises**

Sit straight, not leaning back on the chair, and keep your head in a normal position. Lift both legs up slightly from the floor. Keeping your attention on both of your feet, slowly move your toes up and down. Do this exercise eight or ten times.

For variation, move the toes of your right foot up and the toes of your left foot down for eight or ten times. Then relax your feet.

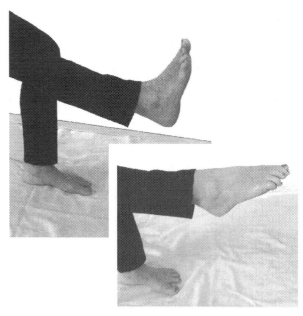

Lift your right foot up and point your toes away hard as you breathe out. Feel the tension on the top of your foot. Then turn your foot up towards yourself as you breathe in. Now feel the tension in your calf muscle. Repeat this eight or ten times.

*Marianna Halasz*

It will take some time to get used to coordinating your breath with all the different body movements, but it will soon become a normal habit. You learn to breathe out as you bend your body and breathe in as you stretch. Your breathing will coordinate with your stretching.

## Rotate Ankle whilst Sitting

Lift your right foot slightly above the ground; slowly rotate your ankle in big circles eight times, and then change direction. Make sure not to move your knee and leg. Relax your right foot, lift your left one, and repeat the exercise (constantly keeping your mind on what you are doing).

Lift both legs slightly up in the air and make large circles with both feet in different directions. Move your right foot clockwise with your left one moving anticlockwise. Repeat the exercise eight times, then change: roll your right foot anticlockwise and left foot clockwise.

Next, roll both of your feet clockwise about eight times before rolling both feet anticlockwise eight times.

## Arms and Legs Together

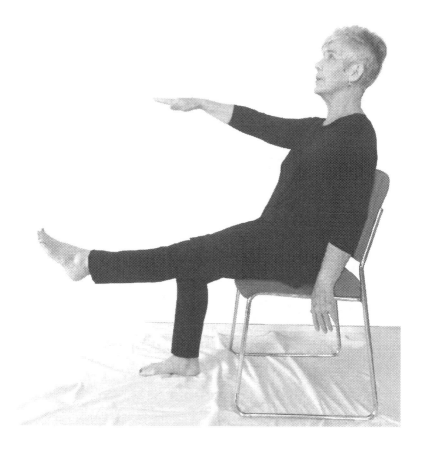

Sit in your chair; breathe in as you lift your right arm and right leg. Breathe out and lower your arm and leg. Then breathe in, lifting your left arm and left leg, and breathe out as you lower them. Repeat on each side four times.

Breathe in, lifting your right arm and left leg; breathe out as you lower your arm and leg. Breathe in, lifting your left arm and right leg; breathe out. This simple exercise will improve your coordination by refreshing your memory and rewiring your brain. Repeat four times.

*Marianna Halasz*

# CHAPTER 10

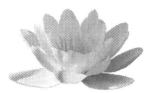

## Hand Exercises

### Rotating Your Fists

Sit with your back straight (away from the chair rest); lift up your hands in front of you, bending your elbows, and whilst keeping them close to your side, make loose fists. Gently rotate your hands eight times. Change direction that your wrists rotate, keeping your mind on what you are doing.

### Hands Bent Front and Back

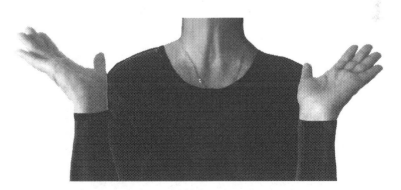

Make hard fists with your hands. Relax your elbows and upper body. Whilst breathing in, stretch your hands and fingers out as far back as you can without moving the rest of your arms. Close your fists again as you breathe out. Repeat eight times.

## Bending Hands and Pushing Hands Left and Right

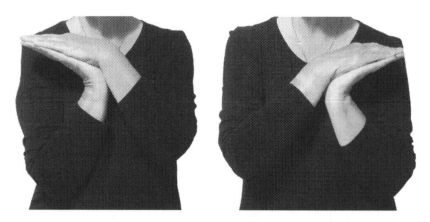

Place the palms of your hands gently together and breathe in. Push your right hand down on top of your left hand, gently pushing your left hand backward. Breathe out, doing the same by pushing your right hand with your left one. Repeat on each side four times.

## Hands towards Your Body and away from Your Body

Place the palms of your hands together gently again; breathe out, turning both your hands downward, away from yourself.

Breathe in, turning your fingers towards your body, lifting only your elbows but not your shoulders. Repeat the two movements four times.

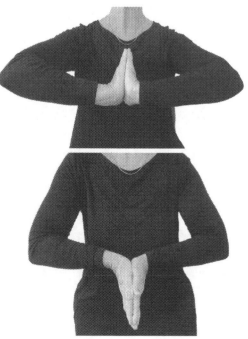

*Marianna Halasz*

# (HAPTER II

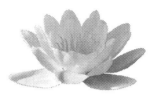

## Movements by Standing

## Sideways Movement and Rotating the Ankle

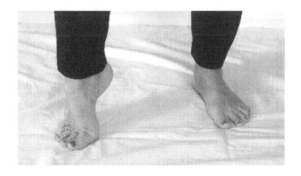

Stand up with your feet a little apart. Place your right toes against the ground, pushing your heel forward. Move your ankles to right and left. Do not look downward. The movement starts with your ankle. Repeat this eight times on your right side, then change to your left foot, repeating the exercise. The movement should be slow.

As your toes are on the floor, move your heel to make a circular motion with your ankle, without lifting your toes up. Make the circular movement four times in one direction, and then change the direction, rotating the ankle four more times. Change the foot, and repeat the circular motion with your heel and ankle.

## Rotating the Knees

Standing with your feet still a little apart, move your knees in a circular motion (think of your knees this time). Repeat this eight times. Change the direction, and repeat it eight times again.

## Moving Your Hip Joints

Keep your feet in the same position as in the previous exercise. Push your hips hard to the right and then towards the left. Do not move your upper body. Repeat this at least eight times.

## Rotating Your Hip Joints

Standing in the same position, make circular motions with your hip joints slowly; don't forget to breathe in and out with every circle that you make. Change direction and repeat circular motion.

## Shoulder Lifts

In a standing position, breathe in and, at the same time, lift both of your shoulders up, so that they almost touch your ears. Breathe out, relaxing your shoulders. Repeat this eight times.

Breathe in, rolling your right shoulder back, rotating it up and front. Do the same with your left shoulder. Repeat this several times, and then change by pushing your right shoulder to the front before rolling it back. Do the same with your left shoulder several times.

# CHAPTER 12

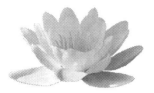

## Head Bends

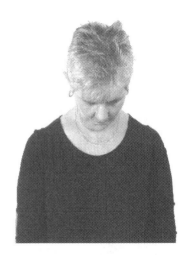 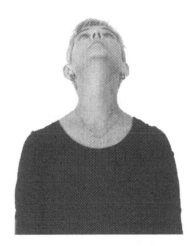

Sit on your chair and relax your whole body. Breathe in, and as you breathe out, bend your head forward slowly, until your chin touches your breastbone. Breathe in slowly, lifting your head and bending backward as far as you can, keeping your eyes open and mouth closed. Bend forward again, breathing out slowly. Repeat this at least four times.

## Head Turns

In the same position as the previous exercise, take a breath in, and as you breathe out, gently turn your head to the right. Breathe in, bringing your head back to the middle. From the middle, breathe out and turn towards your left. Breathe in, bringing your head back to the middle. Repeat this four times.

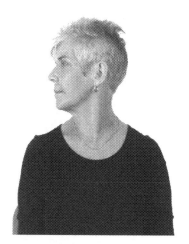 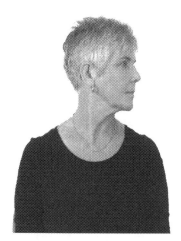

## Head Rolls

Sitting in the same position, breathe out as you bend your head forward halfway towards your chest. Roll your head towards the right and then towards the back (remember to roll from the back of your neck, without twisting or turning). From the back, breathe in, and roll your head towards your left and back to the front. Repeat this roll four times. Changing direction, roll your head towards your left.

The next exercise is one of the best remedies for a migraine or a constant headache. It is also a very useful practise if you are driving a long distance. If you are driving, stop the car, and repeat the following exercise at least eight times.

*Marianna Halasz*

## Head Roll from Shoulder to Shoulder

Standing or in the basic sitting position, lift both of your shoulders up as high as you can so they are nearly touching your ears. Then roll your head at the back from one shoulder to the other, breathing in and out at the same time. Repeat this at least six times from one side to the other. After an interval, repeat the rolling.

Relax for a few minutes. The neck pain or headache may not stop immediately. Having repeated the shoulder turning massage at the back of your head, you have refreshed the bloodstream in your neck and head, and you will find that the tension pain may stop.

# (HAPTER 13

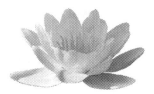

## Stretching and Pumping Your Arms

Standing up straight, stretch your arms up beside your ears and pump them slowly back and forward six times. Lower your arms beside your body.

Lift your arms again sideways to shoulder level and pump them backwards and forwards six times. Lower your arms to your side.

Lift both of your arms up behind you with the tops of your hands facing the ceiling. Pump up and down slowly eight times. Relax your arms beside your body.

## Rolling Your Upper Body

Standing with your feet apart, with your hands on your hips, bend forward halfway; whilst keeping your upper body at the same level, breathe in. Roll your torso to the right and then to the back. Breathe out, rolling to the left and back to the front. Do this three times. Repeat the same upper body roll, starting on the left side.

## Bending Forward and Back

With your legs slightly apart, interlock your fingers behind your back. Stretch your arms, straightening your elbows and pushing your chest forward. Breathe out, bending forward from the hips with your head down, keeping your back bent. Breathe easily for a few seconds. Breathe in, and stand up straight.

With your interlocked fingers and hands behind you, breathe in, and bend your body backward, pushing your head back also (eyes open, mouth closed). Keep your arms a little away from your body. Breathe easily and try to keep this position for a few seconds. Breathe out, returning to the normal position. Repeat four times.

## Bending Forward

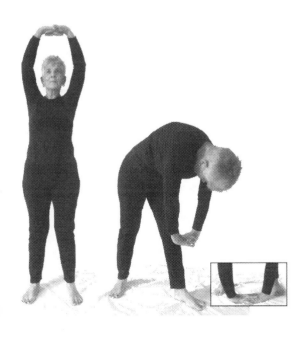

With your legs apart a little, stand straight and lift your arms in front of you at shoulder level. Interlock your fingers and turn your hands inside out. Breathe in, lifting your hands up above your head. Breathe out, lowering them to the front of you and bending forward as much as you can from the hips. Lift your body and arms. Repeat this four times.

**Bending Sideways**

With your fingers interlocked and also inverted, stretch your hands upward. Keeping your left foot securely on the floor, turn your right foot towards your right. Breathe out, bending forward, and try to touch your leg, knee, or foot with your inverted hands. Stand up again, stretching your arms up. Return to the middle, breathe in, and repeat the twist, but this time, turn towards your left. Repeat the process again.

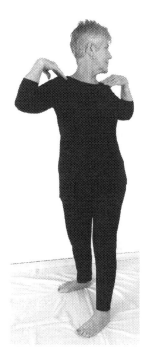

**Twisting the Upper Body Sideways**

Standing with your legs a little apart, place your fingertips on your shoulder, keeping your elbows beside your body. Breathe in. Breathe out, twisting your upper body, shoulders, and head towards your right. Look at a point behind you. Breathe in, and come back to the middle. Breathe out, bending your torso towards your left side. Breathe in, coming back to the front. Repeat six times.

**Bending the Upper Body on Both Sides**

Legs apart, place your right hand on your right thigh. Lift your left arm above your head and, whilst breathing out, bend towards your right side. Breathe in, and stand up again. Change sides. Left hand on your left thigh, lift your right arm above your head; bending towards your left, breathe out. Do this slowly, keeping your mind on the movement. Repeat at least four times.

# CHAPTER 14

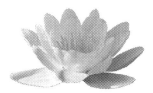

## Sitting and Circling the Elbows

Sitting comfortably, place your fingertips on your shoulders. Move your elbows in front of you so that they touch. Breathe out and bend your head down towards your elbows. Breathe in, rotating your elbows from the front to the back by making a big circle with your elbows. Lift your head as your elbows go up and back. Bring your head down as your elbows rotate to the front. Repeat this rotating movement four times.

Still sitting in the same position, reverse the direction of the elbow rotation. With your elbows in front and head down, breathe in, and move your elbows backward, close to your body. Move them upward, lifting your head, making a large circle, before bringing them back to the front as you breathe out. Repeat this four times.

## Bending Forward

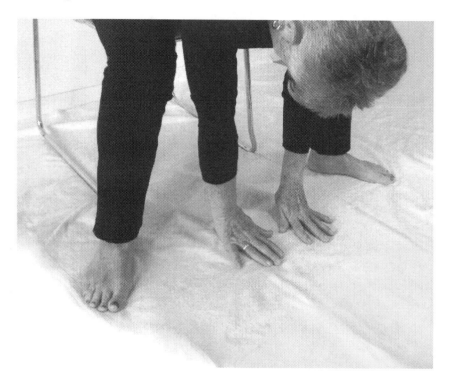

Sitting down, bring your whole body a little forward on your chair. Move your knees and feet as far apart as you can, but remain secure on the chair. Stretch your arms in front of you to shoulder level, keeping your upper body straight. Breathe in first, and as you are breathing out, bend down, keeping your arms straight, with your head in the normal position. Bend as far as you can, but if possible, the palms of your hands should touch the floor. Breathe in, rising slowly up to the starting position. Repeat this six times.

*Marianna Halasz*

# CHAPTER 15

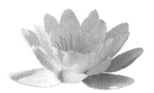

## Exercises to Strengthen Hands, Arms, Shoulders, and Upper Body

All the following exercises should be done sitting upright but keeping your spine away from the back of the chair. Your head should remain in the normal position. Look at a point opposite to you. Remember, whatever you are doing, your whole body is participating. You should always know how your entire body is positioned. Never close your eyes during exercise.

Sitting in a normal position, raise your hands, with the palms touching loosely (as in prayer). Form a straight line with your elbows. Take a deep breath, and push your palms together hard. Hold the position for a few seconds. Hold your breath, and then as you breathe out, loosen the pressure of your hands.

Variation: Place your hands together and breathe in. Tighten your hands, but this time, breathe easily and feel the tension in your hands, arms, elbows, and shoulders. Make sure that you are not putting any stress on your neck muscles. Breathe out and loosen the pressure in your hand and arm muscles.

## Moving Your Arms Left, Middle, and Right

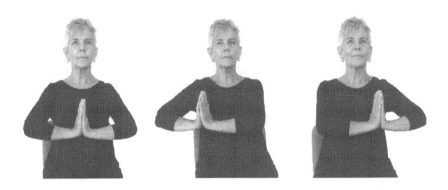

Take a big breath, pushing your hands together hard, and as you breathe out, move them slowly towards your right. Breathe in again, moving your tightly held hands back to the middle. Now, move your hands towards your left as you breathe out. Repeat this four times on each side.

## More Arm and Shoulder Movements

Interlock your fingers on top of your head. Elbows should be pushed towards the side. Pull your hands slightly away from each other. As you breathe in, slowly raise your hands up above your head. Remember that your hands are moving upward, not in front of you. Stretching as high as you can, breathe out slowly. Lower your hands down on top of your head. Repeat this four times.

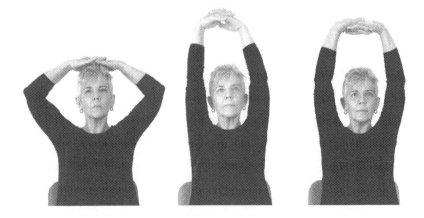

Variation: Place your interlocked fingers on top of your head. Turn your hands inside out, and as you breathe in, lift them up, straightening your arms and keeping them as close to your ears as possible. Breathe out, slowly lowering your hands onto the top of your head. Repeat this four times.

Most people who do these arm exercises for the first time find the movements a little stressing. It must be repeated that you should only do as much as you can. Do the exercises only once if it's difficult for you in the beginning. Repeat the exercise until your flexibility improves.

Persist with the exercises, so that you regain the suppleness and flexibility of your hands, arms, and shoulders. You will lessen the possible impact of falling, as your hands and arms will be stronger. Falls can cause permanent injuries for the rest of your muscles and bones.

# CHAPTER 16

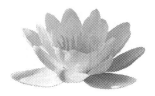

**Triangle: Both Sides**

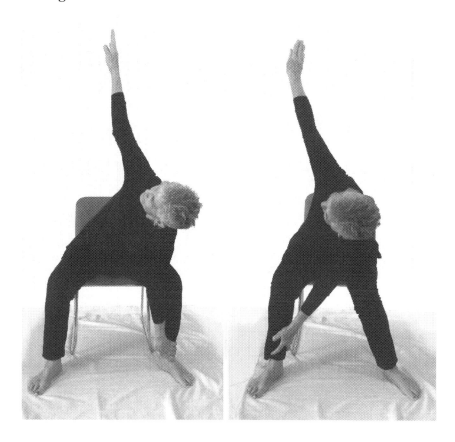

Sitting with your knees and feet apart, take a big breath, and as you breathe out, slide your right hand down the inside of your right leg to your foot. Raise your left arm up towards the ceiling and look up to your hand. Hold the position for a few seconds; breathe in, and slowly raise your body back to a sitting position. Repeat it by changing to the left side.

## Inverted Position

Knees and legs still apart as you sit, take a big yoga breath, and as you breathe out, slide both your hands inside your legs down to your feet. Hang your head and breathe easily.

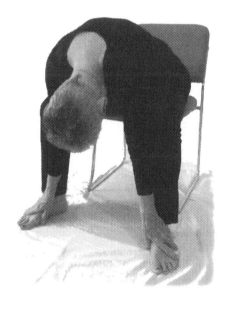

Your position should be perfectly loose, comfortable, and relaxed. Nothing should feel stressed. Hold the position for as long as it feels comfortable. Hold it for a minute or even longer. Come up very slowly and sit for a while before you repeat this posture. If it makes you feel bad, come up sooner.

The inverted position is one of the most important exercises that will keep you feeling young. In this position, your body is almost upside down. Your heart is relaxed, as it does not have to pump the blood up to your head. At the same time, the sensory organs in your head (eyes, ears, nose, and most importantly, your brain) receive all the fresh blood required to refresh and rejuvenate you.

When you hold the inverted position, don't let yourself be disturbed by anything. Turn your telephone off, and don't answer the doorbell. Take your time and get up slowly, because you have a lot of extra blood in your head. If you rise up suddenly, you could lose your balance. You may fall and hurt yourself.

*Marianna Halasz*

# CHAPTER 17

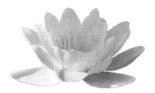

## Eye Exercises

Eye exercises are immensely important. Our eyes give us our vision. They help us to distinguish colours, objects, and distance. Among other things, our sight helps our system of balance.

We can have a long, healthy life if we look after ourselves, with a healthy diet and balanced exercise. Looking after our body should include good eye care. Since our eyes serve us our entire life, they deserve careful attention. This does not take much effort.

As a result of eye exercises, your vision will be clearer, and your eyes will serve you better for the rest of your life. Exercising and training your eyes will also help you to keep your driving license in your later years. If you already wear glasses or contact lenses, this will be really helpful to you. Everyone benefits from these exercises. They should be done at least twice every week.

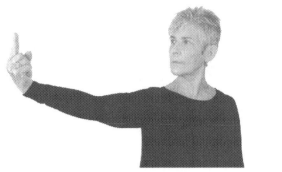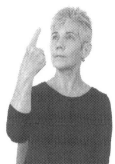

Sitting comfortably but not leaning back, stretch one of your arms forward. Form a fist with your hand, and point your index finger upward. Breathe out, keeping your eyes looking at the tip of your finger, and slowly bend your arm, bringing your index finger closer and closer to the tip of your nose. Breathe in, stretching your arm out whilst still looking at your fingertip. Repeat this four times.

Take a deep breath, and stretch both of your arms sideways, a little lower than your shoulders. Close your hands, and point your index fingers upward. Hold your head straight and look opposite to you. You should be able to see both of your fingers by your side.

Move your forefingers a little if you lose sight of them. Breathe out, moving your arms slowly in front of you, making sure that you see both of your fingers at the same time. Breathe in, stretching out your arms again but looking ahead whilst maintaining your attention on both fingers. Repeat this four times.

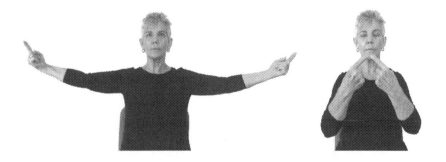

*Marianna Halasz*

Sitting with your back erect this time, move your eyes in random directions, fast. Look up and down and left and right and down and right and down and left and up and right, and so on. This exercise will strengthen your eye muscles. Do this for a minute or two.

# CHAPTER 18

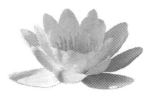

**Standing Exercises behind the Chair**

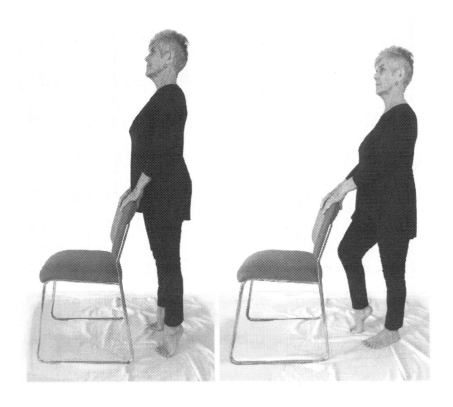

Stand up behind your chair and rest your hands on its back. Keep your head and back straight, and relax your hands. Breathe in, rising up onto your toes; hold this pose for a few seconds, and breathe out, lowering

*Marianna Halasz*

your heels to the floor. After doing this six times, stay up on your toes, breathing easily. Imagine that a string is pulling you upward, stretching your spine towards the ceiling. Breathe out, coming down slowly, and do this one more time.

Still standing behind your chair, breathe in, bending your knees a little, and then come up onto your toes, keeping your upper body and head straight. Breathe out, straightening your knees and lowering your heels back onto the floor. Repeat it six times.

## Squatting

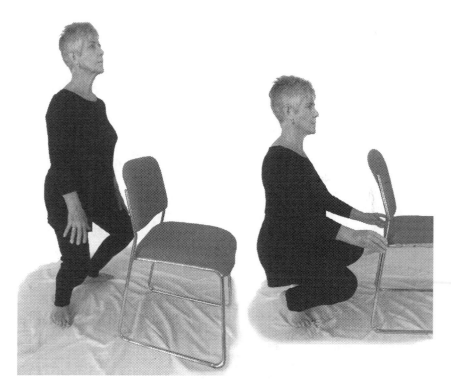

Stand with your hands on the side of the chair. Keep your heels close together, with your toes pointing to the side. Breathe out slowly, bending your knees sideways and squatting down. Hold the position and breathe in, standing up slowly.

As always, do just as much as you can. Bend only halfway (or even less) if it is difficult.

The important thing is to keep your upper body straight. Do not bend forward, as that will put unnecessary weight on your lower back. Do little but try to do it well; if you practise this regularly, you will get better results, slowly but surely. Repeat this six times. If it proves to be a little difficult, do it just once or twice.

Standing straight, with your hands holding the back of the chair, breathe in slowly and lift your right leg sideways. Breathe out and lower your leg. Repeat this with your left leg. Do this several times. When your leg is up, always hold it for a few seconds and then lower it down slowly.

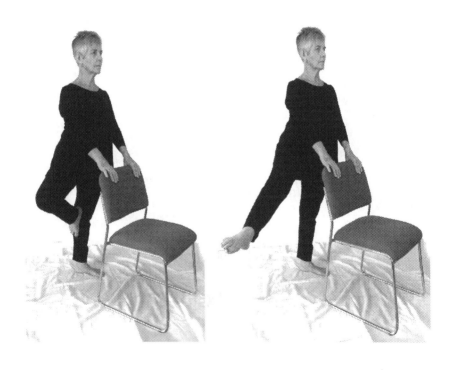

*Marianna Halasz*

# CHAPTER 19

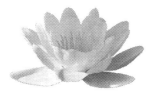

## Balancing Exercises

Standing behind your chair, cross your right foot over your left foot, placing your right toes on the ground. Breathe in, and lift your hands up sideways to touch above your head. Hold one hand on the back of the chair if it helps to keep your balance. Breathe out and lower your hands to your side (pictured below).

Cross your left leg over your right one, and as you breathe in again, lift your hands up. Breathe out, lowering your hands and stepping back into your normal standing position.

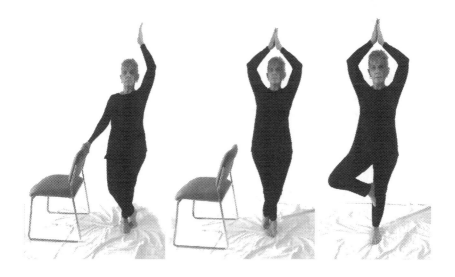

**The Stork**

Breathe in, lifting your right leg; place your right foot inside your left knee or thigh. Lift both hands up above your head with your palms touching, and hold the position. Hold one hand on the back of the chair if needed. Repeat this on the other side.

**The Cat**

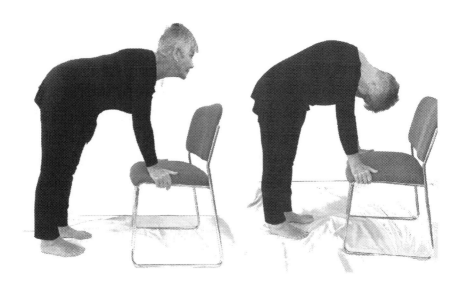

Turn your seat around so the back is away from yourself. Stand back a little, and bending forward, hold the sides of the chair seat with both hands. Your body weight should be supported and shared by your hands and feet. Your feet and arms will steady you during this movement.

Only your head and spine should move, just like a cat when it arches its back. Breathe in, lifting your head up and, at the same time, pushing your stomach muscles downward.

Breathe out, blowing as much air from your lungs as you can and pushing your spine up towards the ceiling. Pull your stomach muscles in, pushing your pelvic bones forward. Repeat six times.

This may seem a little complicated at first, but once you get the hang of it, it will become easy and even enjoyable. The Cat is one of the most effective methods to keep your spine supple, strong, and healthy. Xi, the life force, or energy is moving in your spine. The Cat also helps to align your spine's vertebrae.

When you are pushing your spine up and pulling your stomach muscles in, you are also lifting your pelvic floor, returning all your abdominal organs back to their original position.

This is very important for women who have given birth. Babies growing in the uterus can push the mother's internal organs out of position. So two or three months after giving birth, women should do this exercise to move their internal organs back into the original position.

Men should also do the Cat. Prostate cancer affects many men. The simple pelvic exercises described in this book could help to prevent prostate cancer and many other diseases.

Everyone should do the Cat every day. This would keep a lot of people away from the doctors by preventing spinal injuries. Be kind to yourself, and do the Cat and other yoga exercises described in this book.

# CHAPTER 20

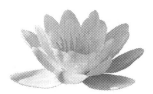

## Leg Exercises

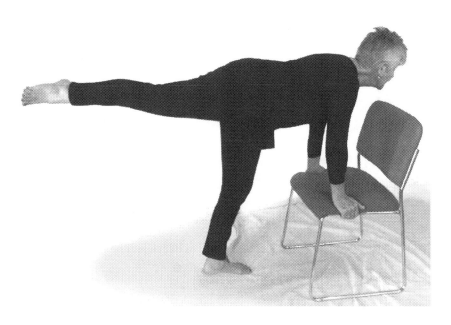

Place your hands on the sides of the chair, holding it securely. Bend your body forward. Keeping your spine and your head straight, breathe in, and stretch your right leg back. Hold it up for a few seconds; breathe out as you lower your leg. Do the same with your left leg. Repeat this six times with each leg.

*Marianna Halasz*

## Bending the Knee Up

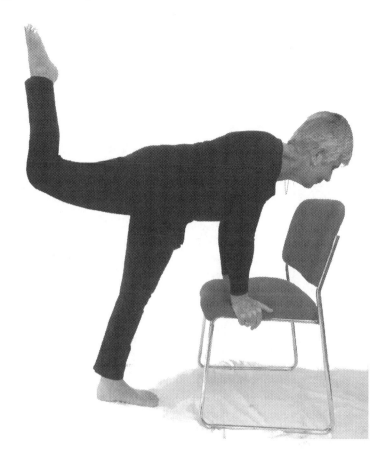

Supporting your body with your hands on the seat of the chair, stretch your right leg back behind you; this time, bend your knee and point your foot up towards the ceiling. Lift your knee as high as you can. Breathe out, lowering your leg and foot down. Do the same with your left leg and knee. Repeat this six times.

Stand up between repeats, stretching your hands and shaking your legs. Always have a little interval between different movements to give your body the opportunity to adjust itself to all the new movements. After a short rest, continue the exercise.

## The Dog Stretch

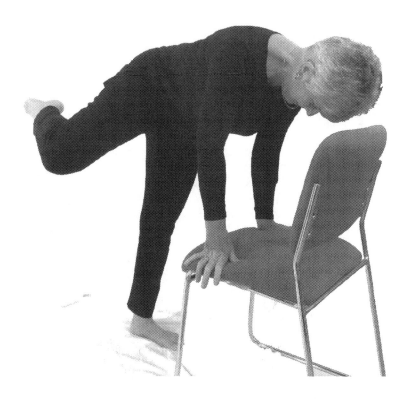

Supporting yourself with your hands on the seat of the chair, keep your back straight, ensuring that your head does not move. Your head is simply an extension of your spine. Breathe out, bending your right knee and bringing it up to your chest in front of you, as close to your body as possible. Breathe in, moving your knee up to the side.

Keep your knee bent, and do not stretch your leg. Your knee is leading the movement. This is an awkward move, but it is most beneficial for your hip joints and spine. Do the same with your left leg. Repeat this six times on each side.

*Marianna Halasz*

## Stretching with Hands on Chair

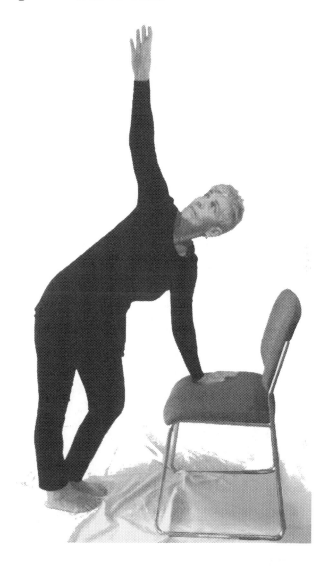

Face the seat of the chair towards you, and put both hands flat on it. Your feet should remain flat on the ground as you bend your right knee a little. Breathe in, as you raise your left arm towards the ceiling. Look up towards your hand. Bring your hand back onto the chair, and repeat the stretch on the other side. Repeat four times on both sides.

# CHAPTER 21

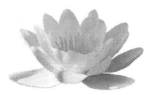

## Kneeling in Front of the Chair

This exercise should be done every day to keep your knees supple and flexible. It may be difficult or painful to begin with, so I suggest that you start by simply going down on your knees (people with knee problems can kneel on a small piece of thin foam).

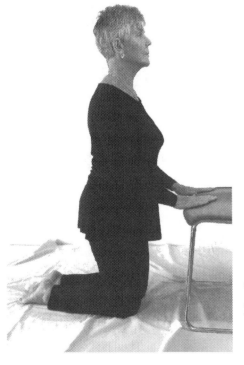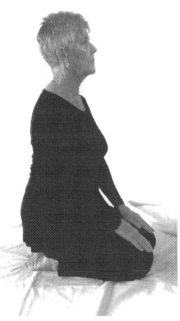

*Marianna Halasz*

In the future, as your knees become more obliging, you will be able to complete the whole exercise with ease.

Kneel down slowly in front of the chair. Breathe in, sitting back on your heels, with the tops of your feet facing the floor. Stay in this position for a while, and then straighten up onto your knees into the kneeling position. Go up and down several times.

**Sliding Sideways**

When you are on your knees, place both hands to your right side and slide your hips down to the floor. Sit on your right hip with your legs still bent beneath you. Come up on your knees again, and do the same to the left side. Repeat this several times.

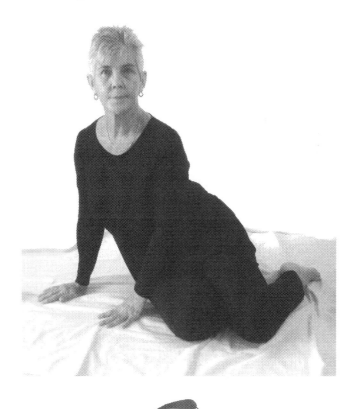

# Gentle Push-Ups

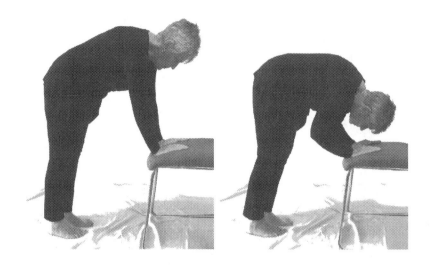

Whilst standing with your chair facing you, bend forward, placing both hands flat on the seat. Breathe out, bending your arms and body (from the hip joint) down towards the seat, with your elbows pointing down towards your feet.

First, make small and frequent bends. Then bend down slowly as deep and low as you can. Breathe out, lifting upward by stretching and straightening your arms again. Do these push-ups for a couple of minutes.

## Push-Ups for the Whole Body at the Kitchen Bench

The kitchen bench, or a sturdy railing, can be very useful for some important yoga stretches. Stand opposite, at arm's length from the bench. Keep your arms straight, and step one foot backward so you are pushing against the bench, keeping your whole body straight. Breathe out, bending your arms and body towards the bench and keeping both elbows close to your side.

Make sure your body is straight. Do not push your backside out. Breathe in, pushing against the bench, and breathe out, coming back to the starting position. Do this slowly at least five times.

*Marianna Halasz*

# CHAPTER 22

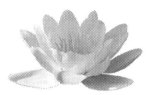

## Spine Exercises whilst Sitting

### Spinal Twist

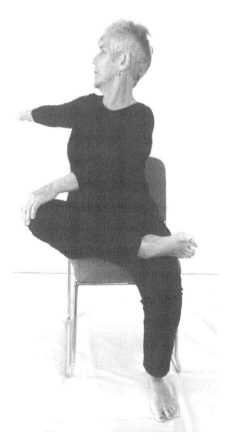

Sitting on a chair, lift and put your right foot on top of your left knee. Place your right hand on your right ankle. Breathe out, stretching your left arm and hand behind you by turning and twisting your shoulders and upper body towards the left.

Inhale and come back to the front. Put your left hand on your right knee; push hard against the knee, and whilst breathing in, twist your upper body to your right side, looking at your outstretched right hand. Exhale and return to the front.

Lift and place your left foot on top of your right knee. Put your left hand on your left ankle. Breathe out, stretching your right arm and hand behind by turning your shoulders and upper body towards the right. Look at your right hand as you turn. Exhale and return to the centre.

With your right hand on your left knee, push hard against your left knee; breathe in, twisting your upper body to your left, whilst looking at your outstretched left hand. Exhale and return to the centre.

### Knee Bends

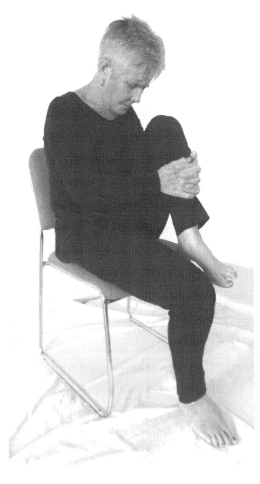

Sitting back on your chair, slide your hips forward towards the edge of the chair, making sure that your body is still secure in that position. This time, lean against the back of the chair. Take a big breath, and as you breathe out, bend your right knee, lifting it up close to your chest.

Using both hands, hug your knee, pressing it as close as you can to your chest and bend your head towards your knee. Hold this position for a few seconds.

Breathe in, lowering your leg to the floor and lifting your head back to the normal position. Do the same with your left leg.

Repeat this exercise four times with each leg.

*Marianna Halasz*

## Leg and Knee Bends

Still sitting, leaning back on your chair and breathing in, lift your right leg as high as you can close to your chest. Interlock your fingers behind your knees, holding it close to your chest. Slowly bend your knees up and down, eight or even ten times, concentrating on what you are doing. Breathe out, lowering your right leg. Do this with your left leg also.

## Leg Circling

Sitting in the same position, leaning against the back of your chair, lift your right leg; interlock your fingers behind your knees. Make slow circular movements with the lower part of your leg, at least eight or ten times. Breathe out, lowering your leg to the floor. Do the same with your left leg.

## Leg and Arm Stretching: The Dead Bug Stretch

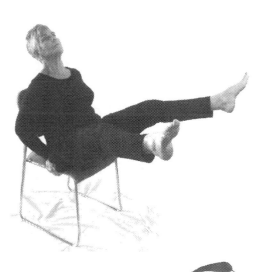

Slide forward on your chair, leaning against the back. Holding the sides of the chair with both of your hands, breathe in, and stretch both of your legs up sideways. If you are able, lift your arms up towards the side as well. Breathe out, and lower your arms and legs. You can stretch the legs or the arms separately.

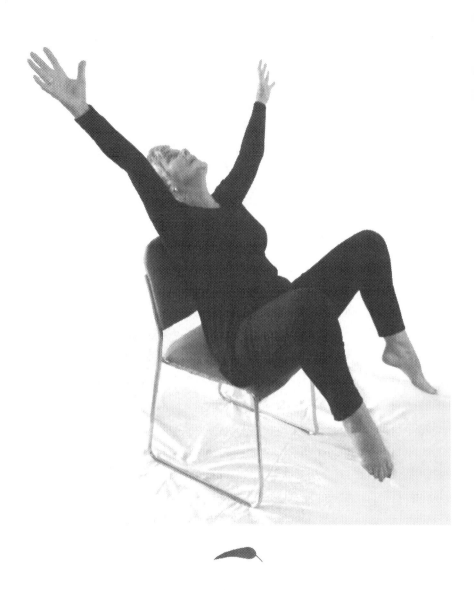

*Marianna Halasz*

## Full-Body Stretch

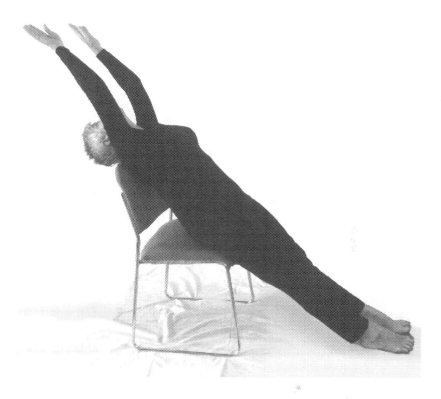

Slide forward on the chair; leaning on the back, take a big yoga breath, and stretch both arms above your head and your legs away from your body, making one long line. You should feel like somebody was pulling your arms and legs in different directions. Hold the position and your breath. Enjoy the feeling, then breathe out and relax. Repeat this stretch several times.

## Body Relaxation: Sitting (Basic Position) and Breathing with Movement

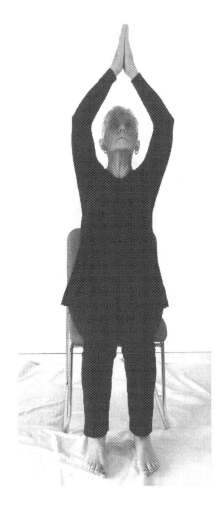

Assume the sitting position with your feet securely on the ground. Place your hands together in prayer position. Breathe in, looking at your hands as you stretch them up. Hold your hands and your breath for a while and look up. As you breathe out, move your hands sideways and bring them together in front of you. Repeat it again, but this time, move your hands and arms first sideways up and bring them down from the top to the front of you.

*Marianna Halasz*

# Sun Salute, Modified Version

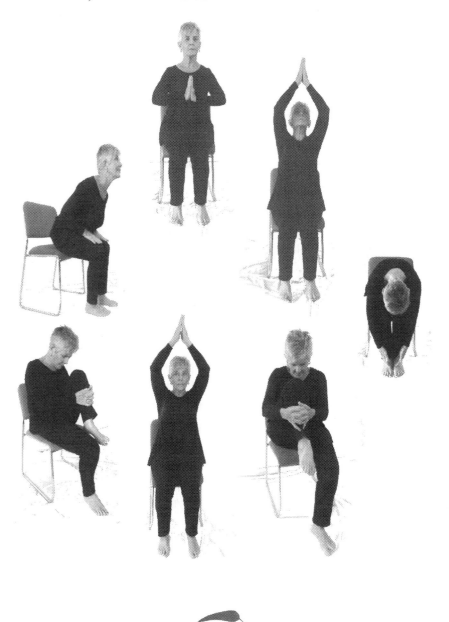

# (HAPTER 23

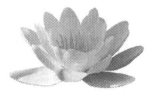

**End of Session: Body Relaxation**

Sitting back in the first basic position, the end-of-session body relaxation is repeated out loud, either by yourself or your yoga instructor. The words are the same as at the beginning of the yoga exercises. The words should make your whole body feel peaceful, healthy, and relaxed.

"Take a few deep breaths, and relax your toes ... your feet ... your ankles ... your lower legs ... your knees ... your thigh and hip joints. Make sure your back and spine is straight. Think of your shoulders and neck muscles. Think of your head and facial muscles. Relax them, one by one: your chin ... your lips ... your eyes ... your forehead and scalp."

The end of the session should be followed by meditation or visualisation, conducted by the instructor. Alternately, a CD can be played. Some very good and calming visualisation CDs are available in specialised shops and on the internet.

# (HAPTER 24

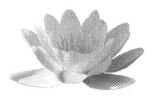

## Visualisation

There is nothing strange about doing visualisation. The word *visualisation* says it all. We practise visualisation every day. We plan and visualise the outcome of future events. During the end session of yoga, we should sit down in a comfortable position, relaxing our bodies in the same way we started our meditation.

With visualisation, you start by creating a certain image. Thought form is energy of the finest kind. When we create anything, it is always a thought form first. The energy we create with our thought vibrations will attract similar quality in our visualisation.

It is best if we listen to a good visualisation CD.

Closing your eyes is good during this time. The other way to teach yourself how to centre your mind is as easy as taking a flower from the garden, a rose, for example. Place the flower in front of you, and give it your full attention. Look at the stem, leaves, petals, and colours of the flower. After a while, without realising it, you will just look at the rose, lost in its beauty and other qualities.

This practise will help you to centre your mind. It also helps you to relax your whole body and bring your whole system of health to a state of balance and equilibrium.

When you listen to a visualisation CD, you are doing much more than just relaxing your body. The trillions of cells in your brain and body begin communicating with each other. The cells will have the chance to function much better. This activity will make you a healthier and more peaceful person.

Make the effort, and discover the benefits of visualisation for yourself.

*Marianna Halasz*

# CHAPTER 25

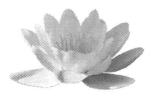

We all have to consider what is important in life. Living in the present and looking after ourselves should be paramount. By doing this, we will achieve peace, equilibrium, and good health. We will be able to project this well-being among our friends and relatives. We can also share it with everyone we come into contact with.

## Meditation

Nobody can teach you how to meditate. It is something you have to do all by yourself. You will discover, after a while, that you already know how to do it. You may have just thought of it as reverie. If you can think, then you know how to meditate.

Most people who have never meditated think that it takes a superhuman effort. However, it's easier than they think. We may have been misled into thinking that it takes a long time. We may also fear that we have to learn something that takes a lot of effort and that the technique is a long process. We also fear that the practise will become a financial burden demanding a lot of effort, practise, and perseverance.

The truth is that meditation is very easy. The act becomes difficult only because we have preconceived ideas of it. We imagine a guru sitting cross-legged on a mountaintop, among other things.

All you have to do is find a quiet place where you can sit down and relax your body. This can be an extra bedroom, a study, a sunroom, a corner of your bedroom, or perhaps a sheltered spot out in your garden. You can use a picture of a flower, a nice landscape, a star, or a respected holy saint as your focal point.

Your choice can help you to achieve the relaxed, peaceful mode you are seeking.

Remember: It is recommended that you sit with your back straight, instead of laying down or leaning back on a chair or sofa. When you lay on your back, your brain's physiology slows down, thinking you are ready to go to sleep.

When you close your eyes, your brain and your whole body system will get the message that you want to go to sleep. Even with the proper body position, it is possible to fall asleep during meditation. It is simply a sign your body needs more sleep.

Remain sitting on your chair or cross-legged on the floor, with your back straight, or sit on the ground, supporting your back against the wall. Keep your head in the normal position.

If you hang your head forward or bend it back, the extra weight on your neck vertebrae can cause a headache. The human head is so perfectly positioned and balanced that we do not feel its weight if we keep it upright.

When we meditate, we contact the deepest centre of our own being. We slow down our whole body and mind system in order to become more peaceful and healthy.

You might think that you are using and controlling your own mind, but the truth is that most of us are so conditioned by our education, upbringing, and the lifestyle we lead that our mind never seems to stop. Our mind, in fact, controls us.

*Marianna Halasz*

"To meditate, you have to empty your mind." You may have heard this sometime in your life. This is like putting the cart in front of the horse. It takes a while to relearn or simply forget this saying. Emptying the mind of busy thoughts is the result of meditation, and not the other way around.

When you meditate, you will achieve state of a relaxed alertness. I suggest that you meditate with your eyes slightly open. When we are awake or conscious, our eyes are naturally open.

When you become more acquainted with this, you will be able to meditate wherever you are. You could be waiting for the bus or sitting in the doctor's waiting room, but if your eyes are open, no one will think that you have fallen asleep.

Keep your eyes slightly open and look at a point at eye level or lower, but do not focus on it. This can be achieved with a little practise.

The simplest way to meditate is to just keep your mind on your breath. This will help you to centre your attention and keep you in the present. This state will become second nature after you've practised meditation for a while.

When you simply think about it, you will fall into this meditative mood automatically. What is more, it will teach you to keep your mind on whatever you are doing. For instance, you can meditate while you are cleaning, cooking, or shopping; it helps to stay in the present.

# CHAPTER 26

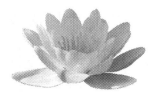

## Sports Problems

Sports can become an addiction if you have been doing them all your life. Even yoga is addictive. However, hard physical sports will eventually be left behind. This may be due to an injury or lifestyle change. If you become sick and have to stop physical activity for a while, as you wait for the injury to heal, it will be difficult to achieve the same results of your youth. You may feel that you have become old.

Even if you are good at a sport you are devoted to, you should also take up yoga.

Firstly, yoga will improve the sport that you are practising. Secondly, after an injury, simple yoga will hasten the process of healing your body and making you feel better.

Yoga, practised over a longer period, enables more persistent bodywork. It will help to keep your mental faculties fresh, active, and young long into your not-so-young years.

While I was writing this book, I received a letter asking for a donation to help an organisation that deals with dementia and Alzheimer's disease. The organisation hopes to find a cure for sufferers. We all know the saying: Prevention is better than a cure.

*Marianna Halasz*

The important question is, how can we avoid getting dementia or Alzheimer's disease? As a person who is still actively practising yoga, I suggest that yoga should be practised by more people. It is suitable for any age group, and it can be done at any time in our life. Good Time Yoga is good for anyone at any age.

Yoga is also an excellent form of exercise for people who suffer from arthritis. The stretches and movements can help to move and loosen the joints of the body affected by arthritis.

Researchers have also discovered a link between constant head trauma and Parkinson's disease. Boxing, rugby, and even football (soccer) can lead to concussion, which in reality is a form of brain damage.

Yoga could be beneficial in preventing or at least delaying dementia and Alzheimer's disease; most members of society live longer, healthier, and more contented lives. We should aspire to become better citizens and serve our country.

Those people who are prepared to practise this method will notice that it is a very good habit. It can become an important necessity in life. It can also become an addiction, a very good one, at that. Yoga prescribed in this book is not just exercise. It is meditation through yoga, or yoga with meditation.

> Between right doing and wrong doing, there
> is a field. I'll meet you there.
> —Rumi

## Advice to Future Good Time Yoga Instructors

Twenty-five years ago, I started to teach hatha yoga. Ten years ago, I began to teach Good Time Yoga for the not-so-young. During this time, I learned a great deal about people and how their bodies and their personalities respond and change through the influence of yoga. The method has also changed my previous perceptions about exercise.

Hatha yoga kept my younger students supple and flexible, using the more advanced movements. However, when I was asked to teach an easier version of yoga, I had to change my way of thinking. I invented the method using standing and sitting positions to enhance the effectiveness of yoga for those who are not so young any more.

Gundagai is a small town in New South Wales, Australia. I posted an advertisement in the local newspaper, and people began to join the classes. Word of mouth by the participants and the advice of a local doctor was passed onto to those who would benefit from these simple and helpful exercises. As a consequence, the numbers grow steadily.

In the process, I learned how to deal a little differently with the not-so-young generation. It is important to

- build up the confidence of your participants, assuring them that they are never too old or that it is never too late to try something new,
- explain to everyone that simplified yoga is just as effective as more complicated exercises,
- tell your students repeatedly to never feel ashamed if they are unable to do everything as well as the person next to them,
- advise your students to avoid comparing themselves to people who are more flexible, and
- repeat many times, just do as much as you can.

The smallest, simplest movement will be better if done by breathing properly and keeping your mind on it.

*Marianna Halasz*

- Explain that the simplest exercises will stimulate the trillions of cells in their body. Cells communicate with each other, and with conscientious movements, they will help the body to gain better health, balance, and equilibrium.
- If someone makes a mistake or does not do a specific exercise properly, don't tell them it's wrong; just explain the correct procedure. You can do this way without humiliating them. Most importantly, never use sarcasm.
- Encourage the whole group by telling them how well they are doing. Don't tell people they are better than the others.

When I started conducting yoga lessons, it occurred to me that my students were actually following what I said and showed them. It was a wake-up call for me. I realised how careful I had to be as to what I said.

Although it is a great responsibility, we can only try to teach, knowing that teaching and learning is a two-way process. Be aware of the student responses, and modify your approach if you find it essential. Try to express your message in a different way.

Think of yoga not so much as a business but as a benefit you provide for the people who need it in their not-so-youthful age.

Don't forget that some students may never have done any exercise in their life, and others may have done sports or gone to the gym, but for some reason, they stopped. It may have taken a lot of courage to start something new and join your class. They may have come to the realisation that sooner or later, everyone becomes not-so-young, but there are ways to avoid becoming helpless and feeble. Your students want to learn how to become flexible and healthy, unlike those who are not doing anything in order to improve themselves. Whatever stage they are at, they should be admired for their efforts.

I emphasise how important it is to be grateful for what you have. This message could be incorporated during the morning meditation or visualisation. By practising yoga for a while, your students will learn how to live in the present, as Eckhart Tolle told in his book *The Power of Now.*

The other wonderful result of doing yoga for a longer period is that the attitude of the participants is bound to change. They won't want to do anything that is not good for themselves or anyone else.

Tell your students that scientific experiments have proven that yoga can reduce their chances of getting dementia or Alzheimer's disease. It can also slow down the effects of arthritis. They will become healthier in mind, body, and spirit, thus avoiding becoming a burden for their family and society. Last but not least, inform your students that those who do yoga feel at least ten years younger, biologically, than those who are not practising it.

Every once in a while, I express my gratitude to my students for allowing me to share my experiences with them. I read somewhere the following line that I want to share with you:

"Do not regret growing older. It is a privilege denied to many."

## Attention to Health Organisations

I have practised hatha yoga for a long time and have taught it for twenty-five years. During this time, I developed an easier and effective method of exercise for the not-so-young members of society. This is how Good Time Yoga was invented.

Good Time Yoga is done by alternately standing or sitting and breathing consciously whilst making the movements. This form of yoga produces the same results as more complicated exercises.

My method become popular and was accepted by people in many NSW towns, such as Galong, Binalong, Harden, Boorowa, Cootamundra, and Gundagai.

Some of my students suggested that I write a book to popularise this method. Many of them also thought that teaching Good Time Yoga would bring immense benefits for all the members of our society and community.

Major corporations around the world have started to hire yoga instructors for their employees. The results are conclusive; the participants enjoy more peaceful working conditions, with fewer sick days and better work performance. The workplace improvements bring immense benefits for both the companies and employees. There is statistical evidence that supports this claim.

Good Time Yoga teaches people how to eliminate the negative feeling of growing old. Yoga, as we know, simply means balancing the physical and mental energy in the human body. With the correct method of breathing, movement, and keeping the mind in the present, longer and healthier lives can be achieved.

It's important to teach this method correctly. It originated in India five thousand years ago; it isn't religious and doesn't contradict the teachings of Christianity or other faiths.

Firstly, it is most important to train teachers the Good Time Yoga method. This can be implemented on a wider scale by future health organisations and the government. Seminars can be organised in every town and city.

I know, from my long years of experience, that there are many people who would be interested in teaching. They would in turn benefit from this type of yoga for the not-so-young.

The seminars for the Good Time Yoga instructors could vary. The participants could be selected from people who are already interested or involved in some type of physical training and have a calling for this kind of profession.

Those who are already teaching yoga should read my book and adapt this simplified method. They would soon realise that it is effective and produces wonderful results.

Former ballet dancers and gymnasts could become yoga instructors. Dancers and gymnasts learned during their long years of training that when the upper body moves, they know where the rest of their body is. With all this knowledge, they could retrain themselves to teach Good Time Yoga for the not-so-young generation.

Athletes past their prime could benefit from taking up this type of yoga. In fact, they should be taught yoga while they are excelling in their professional sport. After their sporting careers are over, they can continue doing this form of exercise for the rest of their lives.

Trainers would need some time to learn how to breathe properly. It is important to keep the mind on the slow body movements during Good Time Yoga. After learning this technique, trainers could teach this method at their sporting facilities.

Implementing Good Time Yoga around the world could produce some incredible results.

*Marianna Halasz*

The benefits for the elderly would be significant. Falling down could be avoided with better balance. This would reduce broken bones and damage to joints and muscles. There would be fewer visits to doctors and physiotherapists. Participants may be able to avoid expensive operations or extended stays in hospitals. Better eyesight could be retained. The onset of arthritis, dementia, and Alzheimer's disease could also be slowed down.

Extended yoga practise could potentially reduce depression and suicide rates, because participants would learn to appreciate what they have by building good self-esteem. Consequently, they would be less of a burden physically and financially to their families and health organisations. This would be better, not only for the elderly but also for the whole of society.

Yoga practise—either hatha or Good Time—also helps participants to feel biologically younger by ten years.

With better health, the retiring age could be extended keeping the not-so-young in the workforce much longer. Highly educated teachers, professionals, and other retirees should be encouraged to teach or tutor high school or university students. This would make them feel good and useful after retirement.

Finally, practitioners require a suitable space for teaching and doing yoga. Clubs, neighbourhood centres, public schools, and town halls, as well as health organisations, have access to larger rooms. Government-owned facilities should not charge any fees, considering the benefits that yoga practise brings to members of the public.

All that is needed is a sturdy armless chair placed on a clean non-slip floor.

Keeping in mind that most of the Good Time Yoga students will be pensioners, grandparents, and even great-grandparents, the fees should be kept as minimal as possible.

In Gundagai NSW, the neighbourhood centre provides the lessons and the facilities without charge, as they offer this service to help society. As a yoga teacher for the elderly and being a pensioner myself, I only charge five dollars per session, per student.

Gundagai is a prime example for all the organisations and Good Time Yoga teachers managing the financial aspect of setting up classes.

I offer my best wishes to all those who are prepared to spread the news and teach Good Time Yoga. This is a heartfelt message; I hope it will reach many people who will be able to make this work. We will all benefit from Good Time Yoga, and when we leave this world, it will be a little better than the way we found it.

# ABOUT THE AUTHOR

Yoga instructor Marianna Halasz was born in Hungary and now lives in Gundagai, Australia.

In Marianna's youth, Hungary was under the Soviet regime. She was educated in Budapest in one of the most prestigious musical high schools, singing, studying piano, and learning music theory. She became a dropout of that school, so to say; it was not her own decision, but a newly appointed principal of the school decided that mostly working class students should stay. So he "advised" about thirty of the students to find another place to further their education. That included Marianna, who was admittedly not the most excellent student at the time; her father was not in the working class but was a teacher of music. The Communists did not accept this background. Among the others who were advised to leave the school was one of her classmates, who excelled in all the school's subjects, but whose father was a high-ranking military officer in the previous regime. Things like that and worse happened to those who did not come from the essential working class.

During and after this, she lived with her mother in a small flat. Part of the building was hit by a bomb during the war and also damaged again at the siege of Budapest. Her parents divorced, so living on her mother's small wages was not easy. There was not enough food and no hot water, and she wore second-hand clothes; they washed their clothes in the bathtub and walked wherever they went because there was no money for public transport. This and other bad things happened to a lot of people in those days.

But there were some good sides of those Communist times. Almost any youngster could practise any kind of sports in the sport clubs, for practically no fees. While Marianna was still studying at that musical high school, she could go to the opera or a classical concert almost every night for a small price, if there were any empty seats. Their home had hardly any heating in those cold winters because the lack of money. But good books were around; a few were purchased, and the rest were borrowed. When a friend visited them one day, he remarked: "What you are living in is a cultured slum."

While all this was happening, she became involved in many physical activities: swimming, gymnastics, and rowing with friends on the Danube. But she was really obsessed with folk dancing and ballet. Interest in the conscientious movement of the body remained with her for the rest of her life and most probably became an addiction. It does happen to dancers and other athletes who compete for long periods.

After the 1956 revolution broke out, she left the country with her husband and two hundred thousand other Hungarians. Australia accepted many refugees at the time, including many Hungarians. It turned out to be one of the best things that ever happened to her.

Her new life offered drastic changes to her circumstances. Not speaking or understanding English forced Marianna to take a job in a factory, which by itself was not bad; it allowed her to be self-sufficient almost from the first week. It took a couple of years to learn the language; earning her living took up most of her time. After she began reading books, her English improved somewhat, and communication with others improved, as did her living standard.

Life went on, and she moved to different locations and had different jobs. In the 1960s, finally using her previous music education, she started singing professionally; for many years, she was performing in many Returned Services League clubs and ethnic organisations in Sydney. Her marriage failed, and it was for the better because it made her realise that she could organise her life and live better alone. All those years and the many ups and downs in life made her body crave some physical exercise.

One day when she was at home, she saw a yoga program advertised on television. What exercise is that? A beautiful Indian woman demonstrated with flexible fluent movement what can be done with elegance and ease.

That woman was Swami Sarasvati. It was a pivotal moment of Marianna's life. She purchased all the books and videos that could be found in the stores about hatha yoga. She taught herself how to breathe and move the body differently. Amazingly, the mind can recall the flexible movements that it did before. At around the same time, she also become interested in visualisation and meditation.

In the 1980s, she moved to Canberra, where she become involved with ethnic groups. Working in radio gave her the opportunity to use of her creativity. The programs varied, including live music and productions by many different ethnic organisations. Meanwhile, she joined a spiritual meditation group and also went to India for a couple retreats.

All these experiences and dealing with restless, peace-less people at work led her to the conclusion that there is more to life than just working and following what other people expect her to do. Yoga and meditation become second nature to her. To deal with some of the stress in radio, she decided to move away from the hassle to a quieter place in the country. After moving to a very small town in Galong, she became centred. She was occupied with yoga meditation and writing articles for the local newspapers.

One day, Marianna discussed yoga with some friends. A few days later, she received a phone call and was asked if she'd like to give a talk about it to a group in Boorowa. She obliged, and following that talk, she was asked to teach yoga there. The news spread by word of mouth that there was a yoga teacher. They asked her to teach in Harden, in Binalong, and even in Cootamundra.

In Gundagai, a friend who ran a spiritual centre asked if she would come and teach yoga classes there. One day, they were talking on the telephone, and this lady told her a house nearby was for sale. This was more than just a simple news; it was a pivotal moment. Shortly after that, Marianna purchased that house and moved to Gundagai.

In Gundagai, she slowly gathered a devoted group of people who first practised hatha yoga, and a few years later, the manager of the Mirabooka Neighbourhood Centre asked her to give lessons for the not-so-young. The participants in those country towns gave Marianna more appreciation than she ever had in all her life. The classes went on ever since, year after year, and she was asked to write this book, *Good Time Yoga for the Not-So-Young.* So here it is, one more yoga book, surely to improve this life of ours on this earth.